15 FOODS

GOOD FOR THE HEART

Unlocking the Potential of Nutrient-Packed Choices for a Healthier Heart

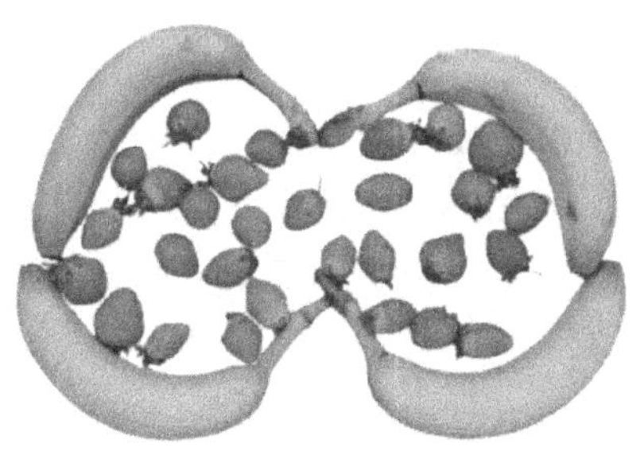

JOYCE A. MOORE

GRATITUDE

This book, ***15 Foods Good for the Heart,*** is a result of countless moments of inspiration, guidance, and encouragement.

First and foremost, I am deeply thankful to my readers for their interest in heart health and for trusting me on this journey to a healthier life. Your curiosity and determination fuel my passion for creating content that can make a meaningful difference.

To my family and friends, your unwavering support and belief in me has been my anchor. You have been my greatest cheerleaders and confidants throughout this journey, reminding me of the importance of perseverance and love.

I also extend my heartfelt gratitude to the nutritionists, researchers, and health professionals whose work has informed and inspired much of what this book represents. Your dedication to advancing knowledge in this field is invaluable.

Finally, to all the hearts that beat with strength and resilience, this book is for you. May it serve as a guide and companion in nurturing both your physical and emotional wellbeing.

This Book Belongs To:

Table of Contents

GRATITUDE..3

INTRODUCTION...7

1. Avocados 8

2. Walnuts.. 12

3. Green Vegetables and Leafy Greens 14

4. Dark Chocolate (Cocoa)........... 19

5. Salmon 22

6. Apple 26

7. Green Tea 29

8. Garlic   31

9. Olive Oil 35

10. Tomatoes 35

11. Oats...................................... 40

12. Beans 42

13. Turmeric 44

14. Citrus Fruits 48

15. Blueberries......................... 52

CONVERSATIONAL QUESTIONS......................................55

CONCLUSION..61

INTRODUCTION

Do you want to maximize your longevity and lead a healthy life? Eating nutritious meals that are rich in vitamins, minerals, and other vital nutrients is essential for your long-term health. Avoiding processed, packaged, and additive-containing foods can help you maintain good health and potentially extend your lifespan. Studies have shown that individuals who focus on consuming wholesome, natural foods are more likely to lead longer and healthier lives. We still influence our health and nutritional choices, even though there is a potential that heredity may predispose us to many different diseases. Even though there are practical methods that may be used to live a happier and more fulfilling life, there are no certainties about how our health might be as we age or how long we're going to live. Below, we'll talk about foods that are good for your heart which will help you live longer.

1. Avocados

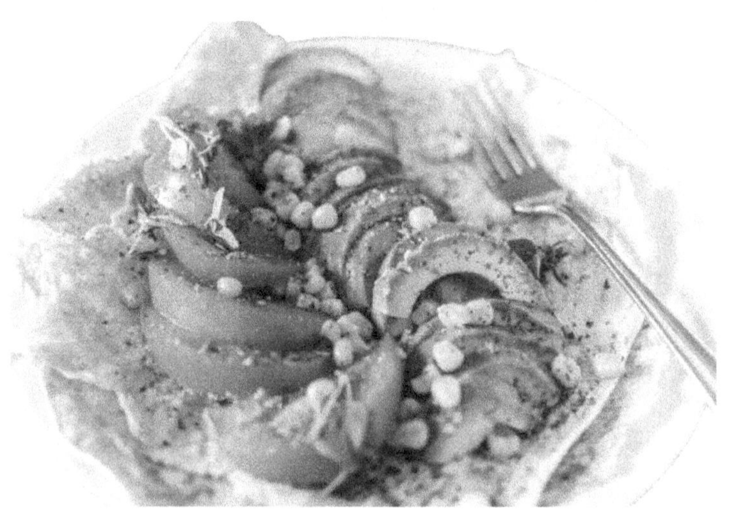

People eat avocados not just for their distinct flavor but also for their outstanding heart health advantages.

Avocados are one of the healthiest foods since they contain folic acid, protein, magnesium, vitamin E, and other B vitamins.

They are also an excellent source of lipids that reduce inflammation and slow the body's aging process. Avocados are abundant in mono- and poly unsaturated fats, which make it simple to produce energy, said a dietician in Washington.

Consequently, blood cholesterol levels can be reduced to a minimum. This fruit increases levels of good cholesterol and lowers levels of bad cholesterol.

According to Reader's Digest, foods with high mono unsaturated fat content can reduce insulin resistance, which helps to control blood sugar levels.

Of all the fruits, avocado's low carbohydrate and sugar content aids in improved blood sugar regulation.

Aside from that, avocados' high potassium content helps in maintaining normal blood pressure. Compared to processed or animal-based fats, avocados are a more readily digested and absorbed type of fat since they are water-rich.

Eating avocados is most beneficial when they are ripe because all their nutrients have fully developed and are most easily tolerated.

In addition to acting as a superb all-purpose food to satiate desires, avocado may also be substituted for fat when baking.

Additionally, you can use it to replace some of your favorite dairy recipes. In addition, it can be included in other recipes such as soups and dessert whips.

According to research, avocado consumption has been linked to several beneficial health consequences, including improved appetite control and weight management.

In 2013, a Nutrition Journal article based on a 7-year review found that avocados are associated with a reduced risk of metabolic syndrome, a condition in which several symptoms are present and may raise the risk of diabetes, stroke, and cardiovascular disease. It also enables better absorption of other nutrients into the body. In addition, studies have proven that avocados can improve cholesterol levels in as little as a week and it contain chemicals that inhibit and kill oral cancer cells, and protect against liver damage.

Although eating avocados has several health advantages, the biggest concern associated with this fruit is that an excessive intake can lead to weight gain because of the fruit's high fat content.

As fat takes longer to absorb than other nutrients, it keeps you feeling fuller for longer, which may also result in nutritional shortages.

2. Walnuts

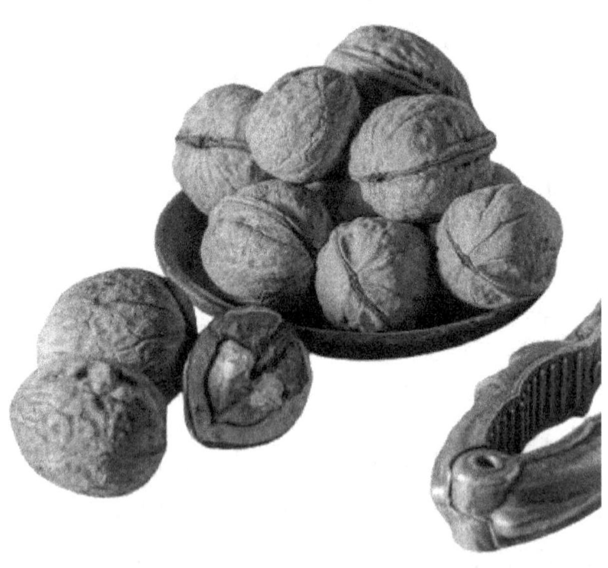

According to a recent scientific study, children who are deficient in the omega-3 fatty acids found in walnuts might become hyperactive, irritable, and prone to tantrums.

A child's mood can be lifted and their EFA shortfall is reduced by including walnuts in their diet.

Even grownups experiencing stress and sadness can use it.

Omega-3 fatty acids can be found in seeds, flax, and hemp seeds, among other foods. The iron and magnesium in other nuts, such as almonds and cashews, support a healthy metabolism and ward off disease, tiredness, and excessive insulin levels.

In addition to having a high fat content, seeds and nuts can assist in regulating metabolism and reduce [AS1] cravings for harmful meals.

Not all nuts have the same nutritional value; some are more nutritious than others, some may include higher levels of protein, carbohydrates, or healthy fat. According to a 30-year study, those who ate nuts at least seven times per week at a minimum of one ounce per serving had a 20% higher chance of living longer than those who did not. There will be a general decrease in the chance of death from heart disease, cancer, and respiratory diseases if nuts are consumed at least five times a week.

3. Green Vegetables and Leafy Greens

Green veggies are good for your heart and are a cornerstone of every balanced diet and lifestyle plan. They are the most alkaline meals that can be found all year long and are stocked with enough vitamins, protein, and minerals.

The greatest leafy green vegetables to eat are those that are high in protein,

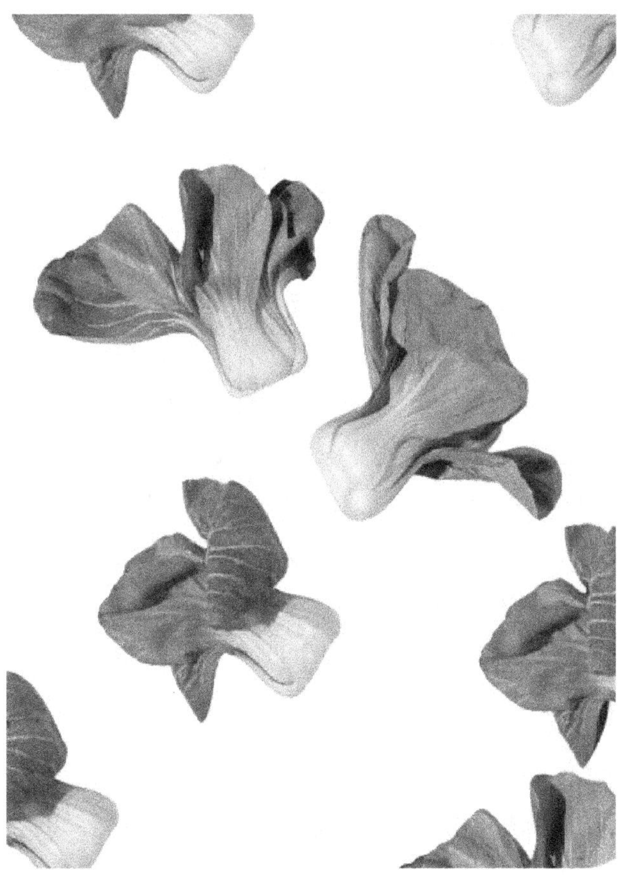

calcium, magnesium, chlorophyll, and iron. Examples of these veggies include broccoli, kale, and spinach. Leafy green veggies also include vitamins A and C, in addition to vitamin B6.

The high vitamin K level of kale helps to develop bones, which is important for year-round activity.

Leafy greens are also among the meals that are the most effective at preventing the early stages of cancer and can even reverse the outcome of some major health problems It is loaded with a lot of carotenoids, antioxidants, and other chemicals made for illness prevention. The antioxidants protect the heart against cardiovascular disease and aid in the prevention of some birth abnormalities.

Additionally, the vitamins in leafy green vegetables decrease homocysteine levels, reducing the risk of heart disease. The fact that dark leafy greens have low levels of calories, carbs, and glycemic index is one of their most alluring advantages.

These qualities make it easier for individuals to achicvc and maintain a healthy body weight.

A balanced diet that includes more green vegetables increases dietary fiber consumption, which aids in bowel health and the regulation of the digestive system which aids in bowel health and the regulation of the digestive system. A gene called T-bet has been shown to respond specifically to leafy greens, according to researchers. These immune cells are essential for the development of immune cells that are found in your gut, which are in charge of treating inflammatory illnesses and may even lower your chance of developing bowel cancer.

There are significant health benefits that those who consume three or more servings of dark leafy greens daily are missing out on.

Vegetables are a varied food group, offering a vast selection and enough to satisfy everyone's tastes and preferences. By juicing your vegetables with sprouted beans, you may improve your vegetable consumption in the simplest and most efficient method possible.

This is due to the fact that juicing makes it simple to digest and enables your body to absorb all of the nutrients found in the vegetables. Cooking may cause the loss of some micronutrients.

According to a featured article, people in their middle years who consume a cup of cooked greens every day tend to live longer

than those who don't include leafy greens in their diet.

4. Dark Chocolate (Cocoa)

According to research, eating decadent dark chocolate provides more than 40 different nutritional advantages, including a longer lifespan.

Since it is manufactured from cocoa seeds, dark chocolate is one of the world's best sources of antioxidants.

It works best when cacao (cocoa) is consumed raw since it has the most advantageous foods that promote a healthy heart and brain.

Furthermore, cocoa's healthy fats are good for you and help decrease blood sugar and blood pressure. According to a 2007 study published in the Journal of Nutrition, dark chocolate contains a lot of flavonoids, an antioxidant class that has been shown to prevent cardiovascular disease.

Furthermore, eating high-cocoa-
content, high-quality dark chocolate is

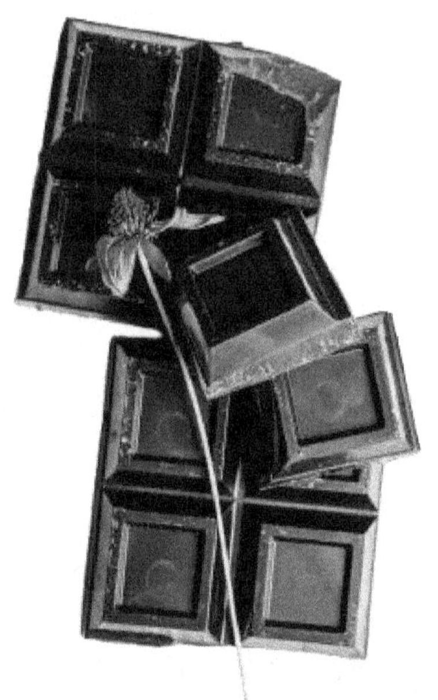

good for you, especially if it has at
least 70% cocoa.

Both raw cacao and cocoa are fantastic
heart-healthy foods that improve
hormone production, blood flow, and
even digestion.

Basically, due to the numerous health
advantages it provides, dark chocolate

is a great sweet snack while also maintaining your health.

But keep in mind that it also contains a lot of fat.

Other than maintaining tabs, chocolate may be the best option if you want to treat yourself. You can also choose organic or raw cocoa powder to reduce your fat intake.

Consuming dark chocolate regularly aids in the breakdown of bacteria and the fermentation of its ingredients into anti-inflammatory substances, both of which are ultimately beneficial to your long-term health.

In addition, dark chocolate promotes healthy blood circulation and reduces the risk of blood clots.

Due to the presence of several chemical constituents that have a good impact on your mind, dark chocolate also serves as a mood enhancer.

It contains phenylethylamine (PEA), which enables the release of endorphins in the brain.

Consuming dark chocolate will therefore help lift your spirits and make you happier.

According to a 1999 Harvard study of 8000 males, those who consumed dark chocolate at least three times each month were able to live an extra year than those who didn't.

5. Salmon

Salmon is not only delicious, but it also has a number of positive health benefits. Salmon is a nutritional powerhouse that is rich in vitamin D and omega-3 fatty acids. It has been demonstrated that omega-3 fatty acids can reduce triglyceride levels and the risk of inflammation, both of which are associated with an increased risk of heart disease.

There is proof that omega-3 fatty acids keep the brain healthy by reducing the risk of dementia and cognitive decline.

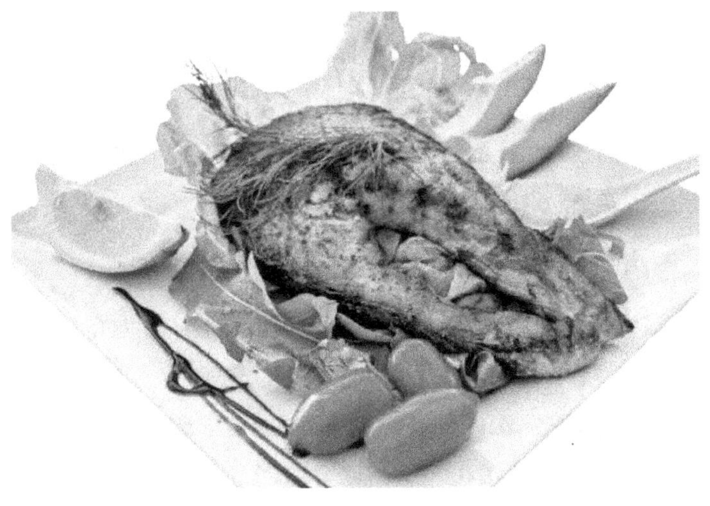

Additionally, giving preschoolers salmon reduces their likelihood of developing ADHD symptoms and can improve their academic performance because salmon's nutrients help kids concentrate and remember things better.

According to studies, salmon's omega-3 fatty acids may encourage weight loss and considerably reduce abdominal fat in obese people, comparing it to the majority of fatty fish, salmon is very high in omega-3 fatty acids. It is a particularly nutrient-dense food choice that only contains a little quantity of mercury, a potentially dangerous contaminant.

Other health advantages of salmon may have been forgotten in the focus on the omega-3 benefits. Salmon's protein and amino acid content are connected to yet another advantage.

Researchers have found that salmon contains tiny bioactive protein molecules known as "bioactive peptides" that can cure joint cartilage, reduce insulin resistance, and manage gastrointestinal inflammation.

Salmon also contains a lot of potassium, which lowers blood pressure and keeps fatty deposits from accumulating in the arteries. It is a fantastic source of calcium, which keeps your bones strong. I recommend eating salmon with the bones.

Regular salmon consumption lowers the risk of cognitive decline in the elderly and lowers adolescent sadness and aggression.

Salmon consumption during pregnancy contributes to the fetal brain's protection and health.

Salmon may be prepared in a variety of creative ways in the kitchen, making it incredibly flexible.

However, purchasing salmon in cans is a simple and affordable substitute that provides the same health benefits as eating fresh fish.
Simply said, including at least two servings of this fatty fish in your

weekly diet plan will help you satisfy your nutrient demands while reducing your risk of developing certain diseases.

Salmon is a nutritional powerhouse that is rich in vitamin D and omega-3 fatty acids.

It has been demonstrated that omega-3s can reduce triglyceride levels and the risk of inflammation, both of which are associated with an increased risk of heart disease.

There is proof that omega-3 fatty acids maintain the brain healthy by reducing the risk of dementia and cognitive decline.

6. Apple

Several studies suggest that including apples in ones diet helps improve longevity, this makes them one of the healthiest fruits in the world.

Despite being the most consumed fruit, individuals frequently ignore their remarkable health advantages.

Apples were ranked #1 among the other foods in a Medical News Today feature article on the top 10.

An apple a day may be the best food to prolong lifespan because it has many health benefits, proving the adage we are all familiar with. First, apples are a good source of vitamin C, fiber, several antioxidants, and folate, which can help prevent Alzheimer's.

Additionally, the peels contain polyphenols, which primarily serve as oxidants. Therefore, it is better to consume the apple's peel to reap the biggest advantages. These polyphenols contain quercetin, a flavonoid that lowers blood pressure. According to studies, eating a lot of flavonoids has

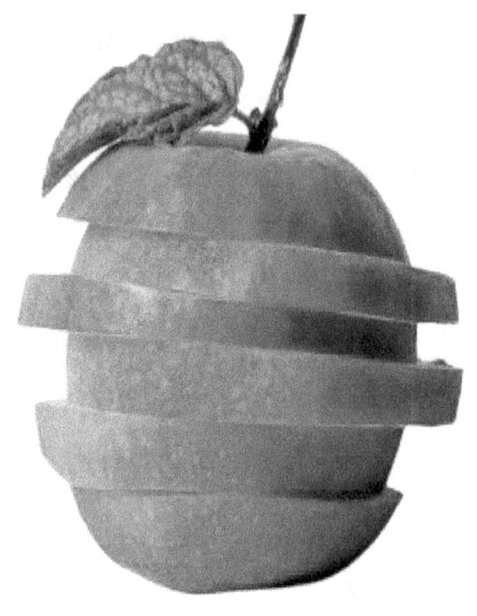

been linked to a 20% lower risk of stroke. It was determined by researchers that eating apples high in flavonoids could reduce the risk of developing pancreatic cancer by 23%. Frequent apple consumption has been shown to have positive effects on the heart because of the high fiber and polyphenol content of apples. Flores further noted that apples have the highest antioxidant level when compared to other fruits, which helps to reduce the risk of acquiring lung cancer in particular.

Another study compares the effects of eating an apple a day to statins, a class of medications used to decrease cholesterol levels.

According to estimates, apples are virtually as beneficial as statins at reducing mortality.

In a nutshell, apples are a fantastic food choice for promoting lifespan and good health because they include several elements that set them apart from other fruits.

7. Green Tea

Green tea is a highly valued beverage that has been shown to have several health benefits, including heart health and general well-being. Rich in antioxidants, this amazing drink creates a cascade of health advantages that go well beyond simple cooling. Green tea's abundant supply of these antioxidants acts as a powerful weapon against inflammation, improving blood flow and coordinating a decrease in cholesterol.

Furthermore, the caffeine included in green tea provides an energizing surge that increases cardiac activity and promotes better blood flow throughout the body. Interestingly, this infusion strengthens cardiovascular resilience in addition to improving heart function.

According to scientific research, drinking green tea on a daily basis may act as a shield, lowering the risk of stroke and strengthening defenses against the start of cardiac conditions. Its powerful qualities function as a proactive move toward strengthening heart health as well as a preventive precaution.

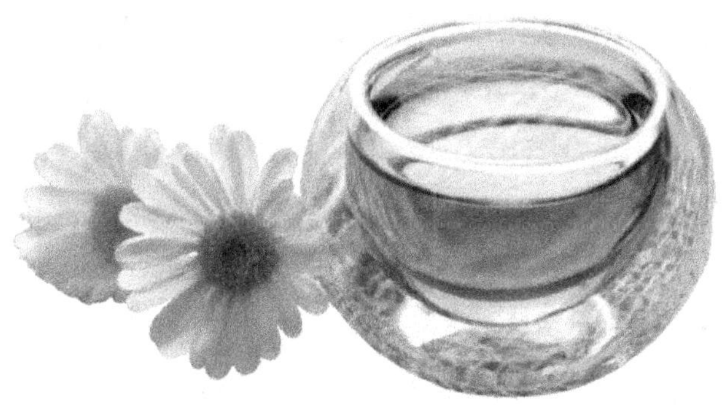

8. Garlic

Garlic isn't just a flavorful addition to your meals—it's a true super food when it comes to supporting heart health. Packed with nutrients, antioxidants, and bioactive compounds, garlic has been celebrated for centuries for its ability to protect the heart and improve overall health.

One of garlic's most well-known benefits is its ability to help reduce cholesterol levels. Studies have shown that garlic can lower LDL (bad cholesterol) while potentially raising HDL (good cholesterol), striking a healthier balance in your blood lipid profile. This is crucial for reducing the buildup of plaque in your arteries, a key factor in preventing atherosclerosis and related conditions like heart attacks and strokes.

Garlic is also a natural ally for managing blood pressure, one of the leading risk factors for heart disease. Compounds in garlic, particularly allicin, help relax blood vessels and improve blood flow, which can lead to lower blood pressure. For those with hypertension, incorporating garlic into your diet can be a simple, natural way to support healthier blood pressure levels.

In addition to its effects on cholesterol and blood pressure, garlic also promotes better circulation. Improved blood flow means your heart doesn't have to work as hard to pump blood throughout your body, reducing strain on this vital organ.

Another significant benefit of garlic is its ability to combat inflammation and oxidative stress, two major contributors to cardiovascular disease. Garlic's antioxidants neutralize harmful free radicals, protecting your blood vessels and heart tissues from damage. This anti-inflammatory action also helps keep arteries flexible and clear, reducing the risk of clots and blockages.

Garlic doesn't stop at heart health—it also supports your immune system and digestive health. A strong immune system and efficient digestion indirectly benefit your heart by reducing overall stress and inflammation in the body. Plus, garlic is low in calories but rich in essential vitamins and minerals, such as vitamin C, vitamin B6, and manganese, all of which contribute to cardiovascular wellness.

Incorporating garlic into your daily meals is easy and versatile. Whether you sauté it with vegetables, mix it into salad dressings, or add it to soups and marinades, garlic not only enhances flavor but also works behind the scenes to support your heart. With its long list of benefits and natural goodness, garlic truly deserves its place in any heart-healthy diet.

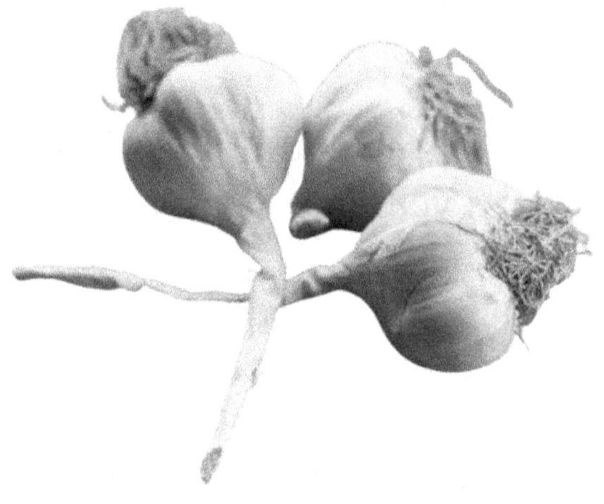

9. Olive Oil

Olive oil is often referred to as "liquid gold," and for good reason—it's one of the best foods you can include in your diet to support heart health. At the heart of olive oil's benefits is its high content of monounsaturated fats, the type of healthy fats that play a crucial role in protecting your cardiovascular system. These fats help lower levels of LDL (bad cholesterol), which can clog arteries, while increasing HDL (good cholesterol), which helps remove harmful cholesterol from your bloodstream. This balance is key to reducing the risk of heart disease.

What makes olive oil even more remarkable is its powerful anti-inflammatory properties. Chronic inflammation is a major contributor to high blood pressure, strokes, and other cardiovascular problems. By including olive oil in your diet, you're providing your body with a natural way to combat this inflammation and protect your arteries from damage.

Another reason olive oil is so good for your heart is its rich content of antioxidants, particularly polyphenols. These compounds help neutralize free radicals in the body, reducing oxidative stress and preventing damage to your blood vessels. This protective effect can help lower the risk of developing high blood pressure, atherosclerosis, and other heart-related issues.

Olive oil also plays a role in preventing blood clots, which can lead to strokes and heart attacks. The fatty acids in olive oil improve the function of platelets—tiny cell fragments in your blood that play a role in clotting—reducing the likelihood of harmful clots forming in your arteries.

Beyond its heart-specific benefits, olive oil contributes to overall health. It has been linked to a reduced risk of certain types of cancer and supports brain and joint health. It's also an excellent source of Vitamin E, a fat-soluble antioxidant that not only protects your heart but also promotes healthy skin and immune function.

Adding olive oil to your diet is easy and delicious. Use it as a base for salad dressings, drizzle it over roasted vegetables, or simply dip fresh bread into it for a flavorful and heart-healthy snack. To maximize the benefits, choose extra virgin olive oil, which is the least processed and retains the highest levels of nutrients and antioxidants.

With its incredible combination of heart-protective properties, olive oil is more than just a cooking ingredient— it's a daily ally for your heart and overall well-being.

10. Tomatoes

Tomatoes are a delicious and adaptable complement to any meal, but they are also a heart-healthy superfood. Lycopene, the brilliant red antioxidant that gives tomatoes their distinctive color, is key to their advantages. Lycopene has an important role in heart health, providing a variety of advantages that help reduce the risk of cardiovascular disease. One of lycopene's most essential functions is to reduce inflammation, which is a key contributor to heart disease. Chronic inflammation can damage blood vessels and cause plaque formation in the arteries, raising the risk of heart attack and stroke. Lycopene promotes improved circulation and lessens the strain on your heart by lowering inflammation and maintaining the health and flexibility of your blood vessels. Other heart-healthy minerals like potassium, which is essential for controlling blood pressure, are also abundant in tomatoes. Potassium relaxes blood vessel walls and prevents hypertension, a major risk factor for heart disease, by counteracting the effects of sodium in the diet. Because of this, tomatoes are a great option for anyone trying to control or avoid high blood pressure.

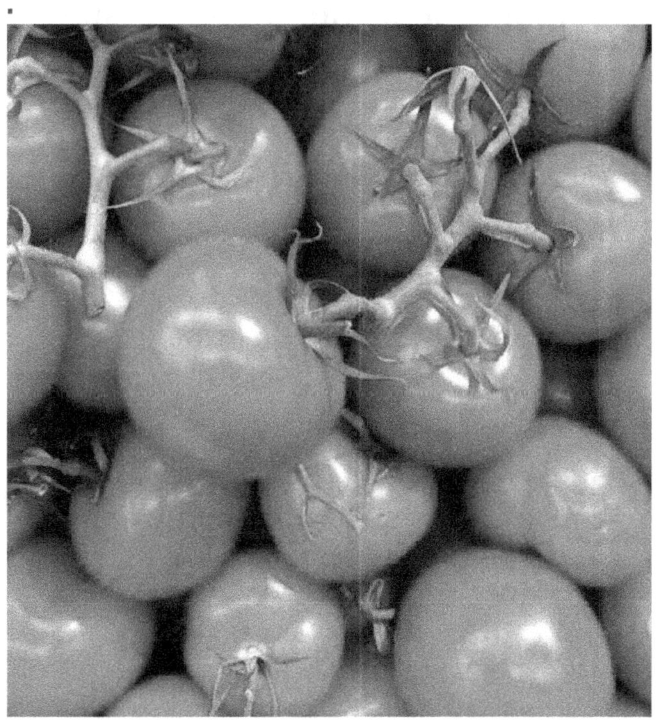

In addition to their anti-inflammatory and blood pressure-regulating properties, tomatoes are packed with other antioxidants, such as vitamin C and beta-carotene, which further support cardiovascular health. These antioxidants work together to fight free radicals in the body, protecting cells from oxidative stress and reducing the risk of developing atherosclerosis—a condition where arteries harden and narrow, restricting blood flow to the heart.

Tomatoes are low in calories and high in water content, making them an excellent choice for maintaining a healthy weight, which is crucial for heart health. They're also versatile and easy to incorporate into your meals. Whether you enjoy them fresh in salads, roasted as a side dish, blended into a flavorful sauce, or sipped as tomato juice, they're a convenient and delicious way to nurture your heart.

Regularly including tomatoes in your diet is a simple yet powerful way to protect your cardiovascular system. With their rich blend of lycopene, potassium, and other heart-protective nutrients, tomatoes truly deserve their reputation as a heart-health superfood.

11. Oats

Oats are an excellent choice for a heart-healthy diet. They are whole grains, comprising the entire grain kernel and containing the nutrient-rich germ, bran, and endosperm. Oats are naturally low in fat, high in soluble fiber, and a good source of protein. Oats include soluble fiber that can lower cholesterol levels, lowering the risk of heart disease. The soluble fiber in oats can reduce cholesterol levels, lowering the risk of heart disease. It also helps keep blood sugar levels steady, improving overall cardiovascular health. Oats also contain magnesium, which helps regulate blood pressure, and potassium, which helps reduce the risk of stroke. They can be put in various dishes to increase their nutritional value and can be cooked into oatmeal, added to muffins or pancakes, or sprinkled on salads or yogurt. They can also be used as a substitute for breadcrumbs in recipes. Finally, oats can be blended into smoothies or used as an alternative to refined white flour. Including oats in the diet can help to meet the body's daily needs for fiber and other vital nutrients for the heart. Eating a diet that includes oats can help reduce cholesterol levels, maintain healthy blood pressure, and keep blood sugar levels under control.

12. Beans

Beans are an excellent food for the heart because of their high fiber content and low saturated fat content. Eating beans can help to reduce LDL cholesterol, which is the bad

cholesterol that can increase the risk of heart disease. Beans are rich in plant-based protein, which can help reduce inflammation and improve heart health. Additionally, beans are a rich source of minerals like potassium, magnesium, and folate, which can help lower blood pressure and improve cholesterol levels.

Lastly, beans are high in antioxidants, which can help reduce the risk of oxidative stress associated with heart disease. All of these benefits make beans an excellent choice for heart health.

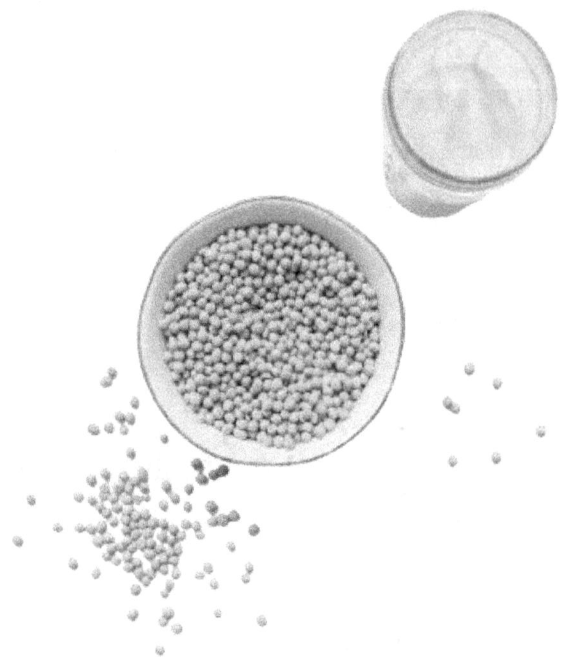

13. Turmeric

Turmeric is a fantastic spice that has a golden reputation for improving heart health. Its potent antioxidant, anti-inflammatory, and antimicrobial capabilities work together to provide considerable cardiovascular protection. One of turmeric's most notable properties is its ability to decrease chronic inflammation, which is a major cause of heart disease. Turmeric protects your heart from harm by targeting inflammation, lowering your risk of hypertension and coronary artery disease. It also helps to improve cholesterol levels by lowering LDL ("bad" cholesterol) and triglycerides, both of which contribute significantly to heart disease.

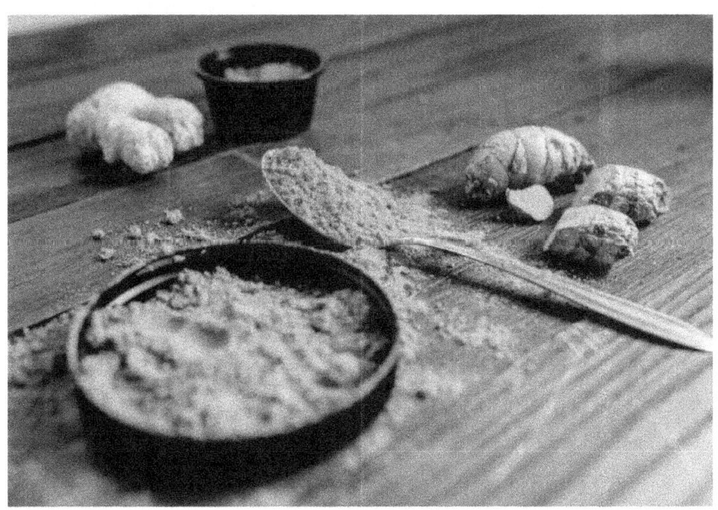

Another method turmeric helps the heart is by increasing blood flow. Improved circulation relieves stress on the heart and ensures that oxygen and nutrients reach key organs properly. Furthermore, curcumin, turmeric's active component, has been shown to improve the function of the endothelium—the thin layer of cells that lines your blood arteries. Healthy endothelium function is essential for keeping arteries flexible and clean, as well as avoiding atherosclerosis, the major cause of heart attacks and strokes. Turmeric also benefits the heart by lowering the risk of blood clots and improving overall vascular health. Studies have shown that it can reduce the risk of cardiovascular events by keeping blood vessels healthy and free of excess plaque formation.

While turmeric is known for its heart-protective properties, its good impacts on other aspects of health indirectly promote cardiovascular health. For example, it promotes liver function, which is essential for cholesterol management and detoxification. A healthy liver helps to manage blood lipid levels, which improves heart health. Incorporating turmeric into your daily routine is a simple yet effective step toward a healthier heart. Add it to soups, stews, drinks, and even your morning smoothie. By embracing this bright flavor, you give your heart the care and protection it requires to grow.

In addition to its heart-healthy benefits, turmeric is an excellent source of nutrients, including vitamins, minerals, and antioxidants. As such, it can help boost overall health and well-being.

14. Citrus Fruits

Citrus fruits are excellent for heart health because they are high in vitamin C and potassium, which are essential for cardiovascular health.

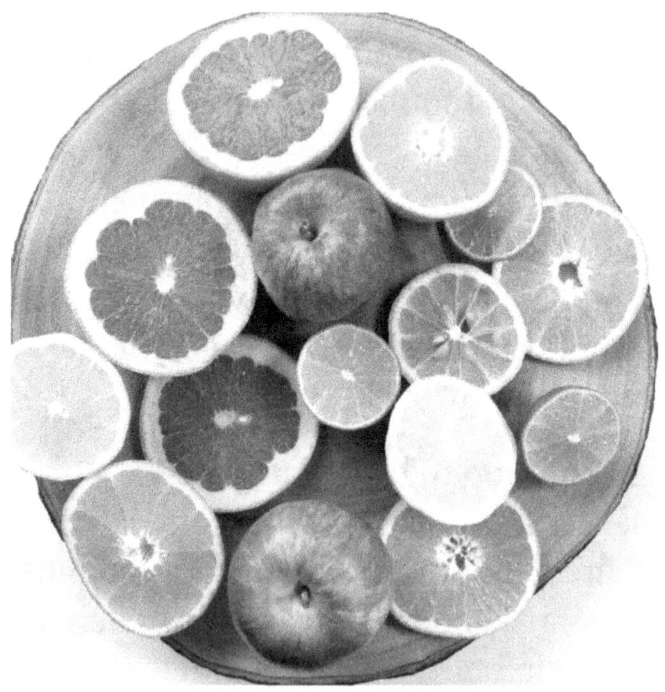

The vitamin C in citrus fruits helps to reduce inflammation and improve circulation, while potassium lowers blood pressure and reduces the risk of stroke and heart attack. Additionally, citrus fruits are full of antioxidants, which can help protect the heart from oxidative damage caused by free radicals

Citrus fruits—like oranges, grapefruits, lemons, and limes—aren't just juicy and refreshing; they are packed with nutrients that can have a profound impact on your overall health, particularly when it comes to protecting your heart. Rich in vitamins, minerals, and antioxidants, these fruits are a delicious way to support cardiovascular wellness and reduce the risk of chronic diseases like diabetes and certain types of cancer.

One of the key reasons citrus fruits are so heart-friendly is their high vitamin C content. Vitamin C is a powerful antioxidant that helps fight free radicals in the body, reducing inflammation and preventing damage to blood vessels. Healthy blood vessels are essential for maintaining proper blood flow and reducing the risk of conditions like hypertension, heart attacks, and strokes.

Citrus fruits are also loaded with flavonoids, plant compounds that have been shown to improve heart health by lowering bad cholesterol (LDL), boosting good cholesterol (HDL), and improving overall circulation. These compounds also help relax blood vessels, which can lower blood pressure and reduce the strain on your heart over time.

For people concerned about diabetes—a condition closely linked to heart disease—citrus fruits are an excellent choice. They have a low glycemic index and are high in fiber, which helps regulate blood sugar levels. This combination not only lowers the risk of developing diabetes but also helps those with the condition manage it better, reducing the likelihood of heart-related complications.

Another great thing about citrus fruits is that they're naturally low in calories and can be enjoyed in a variety of ways without sabotaging your diet. Whether you snack on fresh orange slices, squeeze lemon juice over your salad, or start your day with a glass of grapefruit juice, you're giving your body—and your heart—a boost without overloading on unnecessary calories.

Regularly including citrus fruits in your diet is a simple, tasty, and effective way to nourish your body and protect your heart. Their unique combination of antioxidants, fiber, and natural sweetness makes them a must-have in any heart-healthy lifestyle. So next time you're looking for a snack or a way to add flavor to your meals, reach for a citrus fruit and enjoy the benefits for your heart and beyond.

15. Blueberries

Blueberries offer a wealth of benefits for both heart health and overall well-being. Their richness in antioxidants, particularly anthocyanins, is associated with reduced risks of heart disease. These compounds actively contribute to lowering blood pressure, enhancing blood vessel function, and mitigating inflammation within the cardiovascular system. Regular consumption of blueberries is linked to improvements in cholesterol levels, promoting higher levels of HDL (good) cholesterol and lowering LDL (bad) cholesterol, thereby supporting a healthier heart profile.

Their anti-inflammatory properties help combat inflammation throughout the body, including within arteries and other cardiovascular tissues, bolstering heart health. Blueberries also aid in improving circulation, facilitating better blood flow throughout the body, ensuring essential nutrients and oxygen reach all areas, including the heart. Additionally, the diverse antioxidants in blueberries neutralize free radicals, lessening oxidative stress and cellular damage, which can contribute to heart disease and other chronic conditions. These benefits extend beyond heart health, with blueberries also supporting brain function, aiding digestion due to their fiber content, and potentially contributing to healthier skin. Including blueberries in your diet can significantly contribute to overall well-being, thanks to their robust nutritional content and health-promoting properties.

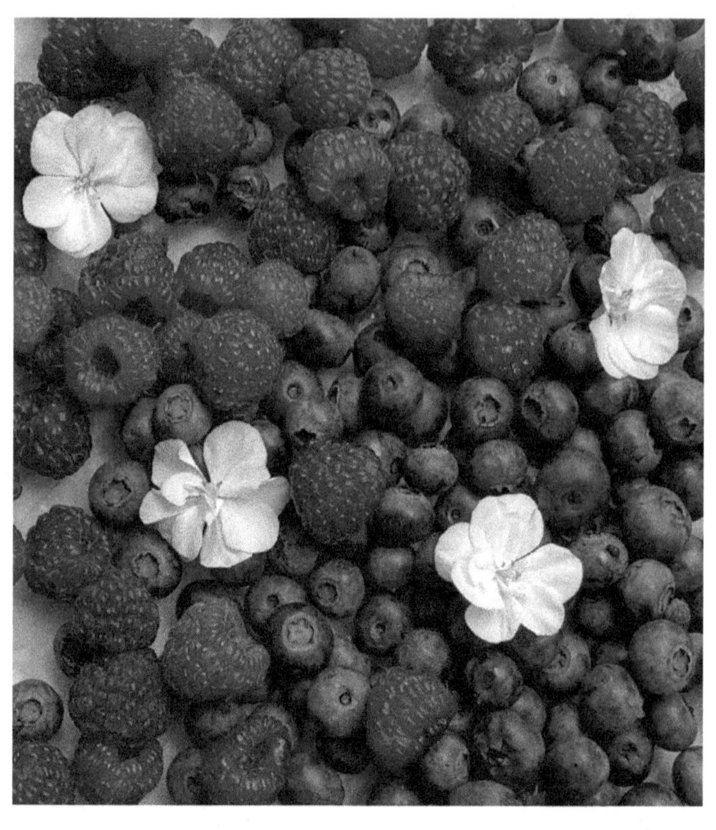

CONVERSATIONAL

QUESTIONS

Which of the heart-healthy foods mentioned in the book excites you the most to try? Have you thought about creative ways to incorporate it into your meals?

Have you noticed any changes in how you feel since including more heart-friendly foods in your diet? What differences stand out to you the most?

Out of the 15 foods, which one do you think might be a challenge to include in your routine, and why? Let's explore some simple tips to make it work for you!

If you were to recommend one of these heart-healthy foods to a friend

or family member, which one would
it be, and what makes it special to
you?

Do you have a favorite heart-friendly recipe or snack idea you'd like to create using these foods? Let's brainstorm some delicious combinations together!

What inspired you to prioritize heart health, and how does this book align with your personal goals?

Have you discovered any surprising benefits from eating more of these foods? For example, better energy, mood, or digestion?

What changes or small habits can you commit to this week to make your meals more heart-friendly? Let's set a realistic and exciting goal!

If you could add one more food to this list based on your personal experience, what would it be and why? I'd love to hear your suggestions!

Do you have a go-to shopping list or favorite store for finding the ingredients mentioned in the book? Let's swap ideas for sourcing these heart-friendly foods!

CONCLUSION

Making wise food decisions can also help you reach and maintain an ideal weight. Start by eating a balanced diet full of fruits, vegetables, lean proteins, low-fat dairy and whole grains. These foods are rich in plant-based proteins, fiber, vitamins, and minerals, which can help reduce your risk of developing chronic illnesses like obesity, diabetes, cardiovascular disease, and stroke. Eating a diet rich in these foods provides a wide range of nutrients that help keep the heart healthy while also reducing cholesterol levels, promoting healthy blood pressure, and reducing inflammation. It can also help you manage stress, boost your energy levels, and even improve your mood. In addition, try to limit your consumption of processed and fast foods and opt for healthier alternatives, such as making your own meals or preparing meals at home. It's important to note that portion control is key when it comes to making wise food decisions. It's easy to overeat when eating out or eating pre-made meals. Be mindful of calories and portion sizes when making your food choices, and stay hydrated by drinking plenty of water. Water is essential for proper body function, and it can help you stay full and energized throughout the day. It is also recommended that you reduce your consumption of sugary drinks, alcohol, and caffeine. Making wise food decisions is just the start of a healthier lifestyle. In addition to adding these healthful foods to your diet, it is also important to limit or avoid processed and refined foods and added sugars. Foods high in fat, as well as sodium-rich processed foods and snacks should also be limited. By making simple changes in what you eat, you can improve your overall health and help prevent certain chronic diseases.

In addition to these meals, there are many other ways to improve overall health and wellbeing. Here are some additional steps that can be taken:

1. Get plenty of sleep: Aim for around 7-9 hours each night to ensure your body has the time it needs to rest and recover. This helps your body and mind rest and repair.

2. Manage stress: Stress can have a negative impact on your mental and physical health. Find ways to manage stress through relaxation techniques, exercise, Take time to relax and practice stress-relieving activities such as meditation, yoga, or journaling, or talking to a mental health professional.

3. Socialize: Spend quality time with friends and family to stay connected and build meaningful relationships.

4. Practice self-care: Take time for yourself to do things that make you

happy and that help you to feel more balanced.

5. Exercise: Exercise regularly to keep your body and mind active. Exercise can help keep your heart healthy, improve your mood, and help maintain a healthy weight.

6. Eat a balanced diet: Make sure to consume a variety of different nutrient-rich foods to ensure that you get the vitamins and minerals your body needs.

7. Drink plenty of water: Hydration is essential for overall health, so make sure to drink plenty of water throughout the day. This can help keep your body functioning well.

8. Take supplements: Consider taking multivitamins or other supplements to help fill any nutritional gaps.

9. Get regular check-ups: Visit your doctor for regular check-ups and

screenings. This can help detect any potential issues before they become more serious.

10. Avoid tobacco: Smoking and chewing tobacco, and using other forms of nicotine can put you at risk for a variety of health issues.

11. Practice good hygiene: Washing your hands regularly, brushing and flossing your teeth, and shower.